# Gastritis Treatment Guide for Beginners

## The Role of Nutrition in Gastritis Healing

By

Calen Bruce

Copyright@2023

# Table of Contents

# CHAPTER 1

# Introduction

## 1.1 Understanding Gastritis

Understanding gastritis is crucial for anyone dealing with this condition or seeking to prevent it. Gastritis occurs when the protective lining of the stomach becomes inflamed, leading to various symptoms and potential complications. The stomach lining is composed of a layer of mucus that shields the stomach from the acidic digestive juices it produces. When this mucus layer is compromised, the stomach tissue becomes susceptible to damage.

Several factors can contribute to the development of gastritis, including:

- Helicobacter pylori infection: One of the most common causes of gastritis is the presence of the Helicobacter pylori bacterium, which can colonize the stomach lining and trigger inflammation.

- Nonsteroidal anti-inflammatory drugs (NSAIDs): Regular use of NSAIDs, such as aspirin or ibuprofen, can irritate the stomach lining and lead to gastritis.

- Excessive alcohol consumption: Alcohol can irritate and inflame the stomach lining, leading to acute or chronic gastritis.

- Stress: Prolonged stress can affect the gastrointestinal system, potentially contributing to gastritis.

- Autoimmune disorders: In some cases, the immune system mistakenly attacks the stomach lining, leading to autoimmune gastritis.

- Bile reflux: When bile flows back into the stomach from the small intestine, it can cause inflammation of the stomach lining.

## 1.2 Who This Guide Is For

This guide is specifically designed for beginners who have recently been diagnosed with gastritis or suspect that they may have this condition. It aims to provide essential information, practical tips, and actionable advice to help individuals better understand gastritis, manage its symptoms, and facilitate the healing process.

Whether you have just received a diagnosis from a healthcare professional or you are experiencing recurring symptoms that you believe might be gastritis, this guide will offer valuable insights and strategies to support your journey towards healing and overall well-being.

This guide is also beneficial for individuals who have loved ones or friends dealing with gastritis. By understanding the condition better, they can provide empathetic support and offer appropriate guidance to those in need.

It is important to note that while this guide can be a valuable resource, it does not replace professional medical advice. Always consult a healthcare professional for personalized diagnosis, treatment, and management of gastritis. Additionally, if you experience severe symptoms or sudden changes in your condition, seek immediate medical attention.

The following chapters will delve into the various aspects of gastritis, ranging from its types and causes to effective healing approaches and preventive measures. By gaining a comprehensive understanding of gastritis and its management, you can take proactive steps to improve your digestive health and enhance your overall quality of life. Let's embark on this healing journey together.

# 1.3 Why Healing Gastritis is Important

Healing gastritis is of utmost importance for several reasons, as this condition can have a significant impact on an individual's health, well-being, and overall quality of life. The following are some key reasons why addressing gastritis promptly and effectively is crucial:

1. Relief from Symptoms: Gastritis can cause a range of uncomfortable and sometimes debilitating symptoms, including abdominal pain, bloating, nausea, vomiting, and a feeling of fullness. By healing gastritis, individuals can experience relief from these distressing symptoms, leading to improved daily functioning and comfort.

2. Prevention of Complications: If left untreated, gastritis can lead to more severe complications. Chronic inflammation of the stomach lining can result in peptic ulcers, which can be painful and increase the risk of internal bleeding. Additionally, untreated gastritis may raise the risk of developing stomach cancer in some cases. Healing gastritis can reduce the likelihood of such complications.

3. Better Nutrient Absorption: The stomach plays a vital role in the initial stages of digestion by breaking down food and facilitating nutrient absorption. When inflamed, the stomach's ability to perform these functions efficiently may be compromised. Healing gastritis ensures proper

nutrient absorption, which is essential for maintaining overall health and preventing nutritional deficiencies.

4. Improved Digestive Function: Chronic gastritis can disrupt the normal digestive process, leading to irregular bowel movements, indigestion, and other digestive issues. By healing gastritis, individuals can restore healthy digestive function, leading to smoother digestion and bowel movements.

5. Enhanced Energy Levels: Constant discomfort and pain due to gastritis can drain an individual's energy and lead to fatigue. Healing gastritis can boost energy levels and enhance overall vitality.

6.  Quality of Life Improvement:
    Chronic gastritis can significantly
    affect an individual's quality of
    life, making it difficult to engage
    in daily activities, socialize, or
    enjoy favorite foods. By healing
    gastritis, individuals can regain
    control of their lives and enjoy a
    higher quality of life.

7.  Reduction of Stress and Anxiety:
    Living with gastritis can be
    emotionally challenging, causing
    stress and anxiety related to the
    uncertainty of symptoms and
    potential complications. Healing
    gastritis can alleviate these
    emotional burdens and promote a
    sense of well-being.

8.  Avoidance of Medication Side
    Effects: While medical treatment
    may be necessary in some cases, it
    often involves the use of

medications that can have side effects. By healing gastritis naturally, individuals may reduce their reliance on medications and avoid potential adverse reactions.

9. Long-Term Digestive Health: Taking proactive steps to heal gastritis can contribute to long-term digestive health. By identifying triggers and adopting a healthier lifestyle, individuals can reduce the likelihood of gastritis recurrence and other digestive issues.

10. Overall Wellness: The health of the digestive system is closely linked to overall wellness. Healing gastritis not only improves gastrointestinal health but also has a positive impact on the immune system, mental health, and various other aspects of well-being.

Healing gastritis is essential to alleviate symptoms, prevent complications, improve digestion, enhance overall well-being, and maintain long-term digestive health. By understanding the importance of addressing gastritis promptly and adopting appropriate healing strategies, individuals can embark on a journey towards better health and a higher quality of life.

# CHAPTER 2

# Types and Causes of Gastritis

## 2.1 Acute Gastritis

Acute gastritis is a sudden and temporary inflammation of the stomach lining. It develops rapidly and is often characterized by the sudden onset of symptoms. While it can be uncomfortable and cause digestive disturbances, acute gastritis typically resolves within a short period, especially with appropriate management. The following are common causes of acute gastritis:

1.  Helicobacter pylori Infection: The Helicobacter pylori bacterium is a primary cause of acute gastritis.

This infection can lead to the rapid onset of inflammation in the stomach lining. Helicobacter pylori is a common bacterial infection worldwide and is often transmitted through contaminated food, water, or person-to-person contact.

2. Nonsteroidal Anti-Inflammatory Drugs (NSAIDs): Frequent or prolonged use of NSAIDs, such as aspirin, ibuprofen, and naproxen, can irritate the stomach lining and trigger acute gastritis. These medications are commonly used for pain relief and to reduce inflammation, but they can cause gastrointestinal side effects.

3. Excessive Alcohol Consumption: Drinking excessive amounts of alcohol can irritate and inflame the stomach lining, leading to acute

gastritis. Alcohol can increase
stomach acid production and
impair the protective mucus layer,
making the stomach more
vulnerable to damage.

4.  Stress: Acute gastritis can
    sometimes be triggered or
    exacerbated by stress. Stress
    activates the body's "fight or
    flight" response, which can affect
    digestive processes and increase
    the risk of inflammation in the
    stomach lining.

5.  Food Poisoning: Ingestion of
    contaminated food or water
    containing harmful bacteria or
    toxins can lead to acute gastritis.
    Food poisoning can cause sudden
    and severe inflammation of the
    stomach lining, along with other
    gastrointestinal symptoms.

6. Viral Infections: Certain viral infections, such as the herpes simplex virus or cytomegalovirus, can cause acute gastritis in some cases.

Treatment for acute gastritis typically focuses on addressing the underlying cause, alleviating symptoms, and allowing the stomach lining to heal. This may involve discontinuing NSAIDs, treating Helicobacter pylori infection with antibiotics, avoiding alcohol and irritants, and implementing a bland diet to reduce stomach irritation.

## 2.2 Chronic Gastritis

Chronic gastritis is a long-term inflammation of the stomach lining that persists for an extended period, often for months or years. Unlike acute gastritis, chronic gastritis develops gradually and may not present noticeable symptoms in its early stages. The following are common causes of chronic gastritis:

1. Helicobacter pylori Infection: Chronic gastritis is commonly associated with a long-term Helicobacter pylori infection. If left untreated, the bacterium can persist in the stomach lining, leading to ongoing inflammation.

2. Autoimmune Disorders: In some cases, chronic gastritis is caused by an autoimmune response in which the immune system mistakenly attacks the stomach lining cells. This condition is known as autoimmune gastritis and may lead to reduced production of stomach acid and

intrinsic factor, essential for vitamin B12 absorption.

3.  Pernicious Anemia: Chronic gastritis can lead to a condition called pernicious anemia, where the body cannot properly absorb vitamin B12 due to the lack of intrinsic factor. This can result from autoimmune gastritis or other factors affecting intrinsic factor production.

4.  Bile Reflux: Chronic bile reflux, where bile flows back into the stomach from the small intestine, can irritate the stomach lining and lead to ongoing inflammation.

5.  Chronic Use of NSAIDs: Long-term and frequent use of NSAIDs can contribute to chronic gastritis, as these medications can

continuously irritate the stomach lining.

6. Environmental and Lifestyle Factors: Smoking, excessive alcohol consumption, and a diet high in spicy or acidic foods can contribute to chronic gastritis.

Treatment for chronic gastritis aims to manage symptoms, reduce inflammation, and prevent complications. Treatment strategies may include the use of acid-reducing medications, antibiotics to treat Helicobacter pylori infection, vitamin B12 supplementation, and dietary modifications.

It is essential to diagnose the specific cause of chronic gastritis to tailor the treatment approach accordingly. Additionally, long-term management may involve lifestyle changes to reduce triggers and support the healing of the stomach lining. Regular follow-up with a healthcare professional is crucial to monitor the condition's progress and adjust the treatment plan as needed.

## 2.3 Common Causes of Gastritis

Gastritis can have various causes, and identifying the underlying factors is essential for effective management and healing. While some causes of gastritis are acute and easily treatable, others may lead to chronic inflammation. The following are common causes of gastritis:

1.  Helicobacter pylori Infection: This bacterium is one of the most prevalent causes of both acute and

chronic gastritis. Helicobacter pylori infects the stomach lining, leading to inflammation and potential complications if left untreated.

2. Nonsteroidal Anti-Inflammatory Drugs (NSAIDs): Frequent or prolonged use of NSAIDs, such as aspirin, ibuprofen, and naproxen, can irritate the stomach lining and cause gastritis. These medications can disrupt the stomach's protective mucus layer, making it susceptible to damage.

3. Excessive Alcohol Consumption: Consuming large amounts of alcohol can irritate and inflame the stomach lining, leading to acute or chronic gastritis. Chronic alcohol consumption can be particularly damaging to the stomach lining.

4. Stress and Anxiety: Prolonged stress can impact the digestive system and increase the risk of gastritis. Stress triggers the release of certain hormones that affect stomach acid production and blood flow to the stomach lining.

5. Autoimmune Disorders: In cases of autoimmune gastritis, the immune system mistakenly attacks the cells of the stomach lining, leading to chronic inflammation. This condition can be associated with reduced production of stomach acid and intrinsic factor, which can affect nutrient absorption.

6. Bile Reflux: When bile flows back into the stomach from the small intestine, it can irritate the stomach lining and cause gastritis. Bile reflux can be caused by conditions

such as bile reflux disease or surgery involving the removal of the gallbladder.

7. Viral Infections: Certain viral infections, such as herpes simplex virus or cytomegalovirus, can cause acute gastritis in some cases.

8. Environmental and Lifestyle Factors: Smoking, eating a diet high in spicy or acidic foods, and consuming caffeine may contribute to gastritis or exacerbate existing inflammation.

## 2.4 Identifying Triggers

Identifying triggers for gastritis is essential to effectively manage and prevent recurrent episodes. Here are some strategies to identify potential triggers:

1.  Keep a Food Diary: Keeping a
    record of the foods you consume
    and any symptoms experienced
    afterward can help identify dietary
    triggers. Note down what you eat,
    the portion sizes, and the time of
    day. Look for patterns between
    specific foods or food groups and
    the occurrence or worsening of
    gastritis symptoms.

2.  Monitor Medication Use: If you
    take NSAIDs or other medications
    regularly, discuss their usage with
    your healthcare provider. They
    may suggest alternative pain relief
    methods or prescribe stomach-
    protective medications if NSAIDs
    are necessary.

3.  Test for Helicobacter pylori: If
    gastritis is suspected, a healthcare
    professional may recommend a
    test for Helicobacter pylori

infection. This may involve a breath test, blood test, or stool test to detect the presence of the bacterium.

4. Evaluate Lifestyle Factors: Assess lifestyle habits, such as alcohol consumption, smoking, and stress levels, to determine if any of these factors may be contributing to gastritis.

5. Monitor Stress Levels: Pay attention to your stress levels and how they correlate with gastritis symptoms. Engage in stress-reducing activities, such as meditation, yoga, or exercise, to help manage stress.

6. Seek Professional Guidance: If you are unsure about the cause of your gastritis or need help identifying triggers, consult a

healthcare professional. They can perform tests, review your medical history, and provide personalized guidance to manage and prevent gastritis.

By identifying and addressing potential triggers, individuals can effectively manage gastritis and take proactive steps to prevent its recurrence. It is essential to work closely with a healthcare provider to develop a comprehensive treatment plan and make necessary lifestyle adjustments for long-term digestive health.

# CHAPTER 2

# Recognizing Gastritis Symptoms

## 3.1 Common Signs and Symptoms

Gastritis can present with a range of signs and symptoms, which can vary in intensity and duration depending on the underlying cause and the type of gastritis (acute or chronic). Not everyone with gastritis will experience all of these symptoms, and some individuals may have mild or no symptoms at all. It is crucial to pay attention to any unusual or persistent digestive issues and seek medical evaluation if needed. Here are some common signs and symptoms of gastritis:

1. Abdominal Pain: The most common symptom of gastritis is abdominal pain or discomfort. It may be described as a dull, gnawing ache or a burning sensation in the upper abdomen. The pain can be intermittent or constant and may worsen after eating certain foods or during times of stress.

2. Nausea and Vomiting: Gastritis can cause feelings of nausea and may lead to vomiting in some cases. Vomiting may be more frequent in acute gastritis, especially if it is caused by infections or irritants.

3. Bloating and Gas: Gastritis can contribute to excessive gas and

bloating, leading to discomfort and a feeling of fullness in the abdomen.

4. Loss of Appetite: Some individuals with gastritis may experience a decreased appetite due to the discomfort associated with eating or as a result of nausea.

5. Indigestion: Gastritis can cause indigestion or dyspepsia, characterized by a feeling of discomfort or heaviness in the upper abdomen after eating.

6. Belching: Excessive belching or burping may occur in some individuals with gastritis, especially if there is an excess buildup of gas in the stomach.

7. Heartburn: Gastritis can lead to a burning sensation or discomfort in the chest, commonly referred to as

heartburn. This symptom may be more pronounced in cases of chronic gastritis.

8. Black or Tarry Stools: In some cases, gastritis can cause bleeding in the stomach, resulting in the passage of black or tarry stools, indicating the presence of digested blood. This is known as melena and requires immediate medical attention.

9. Fatigue: Chronic gastritis, especially if it leads to vitamin deficiencies (e.g., vitamin B12 deficiency due to impaired absorption), can cause fatigue and weakness.

10. Unintended Weight Loss: Persistent gastritis, particularly when accompanied by loss of

appetite and malabsorption issues,
can lead to unintended weight loss.

It is essential to note that some of these symptoms may overlap with other gastrointestinal conditions, making the diagnosis of gastritis more challenging. Additionally, some individuals may have asymptomatic gastritis, where there are no noticeable symptoms despite the presence of inflammation in the stomach lining. If you experience any of these symptoms persistently or have concerns about your digestive health, consult a healthcare professional for proper evaluation and diagnosis. Early detection and appropriate management of gastritis can help prevent complications and promote healing.

## 3.2 When to Seek Medical Help

Knowing when to seek medical help for gastritis is crucial to ensure timely diagnosis, appropriate treatment, and prevention of potential complications. While mild and acute gastritis may resolve on its own or with home remedies, certain situations warrant immediate medical attention. Here are some guidelines for when to seek medical help for gastritis:

1. Persistent or Severe Symptoms: If you experience persistent or severe symptoms of gastritis, such as intense abdominal pain, recurrent vomiting, or signs of dehydration (e.g., extreme thirst, dry mouth, dark urine), seek medical help promptly.

2.  Black or Tarry Stools: The passage
    of black or tarry stools, known as
    melena, may indicate bleeding in
    the digestive tract. If you notice
    this symptom, it is a medical
    emergency, and you should seek
    immediate attention.

3.  Vomiting Blood: If you vomit
    blood or material that resembles
    coffee grounds, it suggests
    bleeding in the upper
    gastrointestinal tract. This requires
    immediate medical attention.

4.  Difficulty Swallowing: If you
    experience difficulty swallowing
    or a feeling of food getting stuck in
    your throat, it may indicate more
    severe inflammation or a structural
    issue. Seek medical help if this
    occurs.

5. Frequent Recurrence of Symptoms: If you have a history of recurrent or chronic gastritis, and your symptoms worsen or return frequently, it is essential to consult a healthcare professional for further evaluation and management.

6. Unintended Weight Loss: Significant and unexplained weight loss without a change in diet or exercise habits should prompt medical evaluation to rule out underlying health issues, including chronic gastritis.

7. Presence of Chronic Health Conditions: If you have pre-existing health conditions such as autoimmune disorders or a history of stomach ulcers, it is crucial to consult a healthcare professional

promptly if you experience new or worsening digestive symptoms.

8.  Medication Side Effects: If you are taking medications known to irritate the stomach lining (e.g., NSAIDs) and experience gastrointestinal symptoms, discuss this with your healthcare professional to explore alternative treatment options.

9.  Suspected Helicobacter pylori Infection: If you suspect or have been informed of a Helicobacter pylori infection, it is essential to seek medical evaluation and treatment to prevent gastritis complications and further health issues.

10. Severe Pain or Discomfort: If you experience severe or unrelenting abdominal pain or discomfort,

especially in the upper abdomen, do not hesitate to seek medical attention.

Early intervention and appropriate medical care can prevent gastritis from progressing to more severe forms or causing long-term complications. If you are unsure whether your symptoms warrant medical attention, it is always best to err on the side of caution and consult a healthcare professional. They can provide proper evaluation, diagnosis, and guidance for managing gastritis effectively and promoting digestive health.

# CHAPTER 4

# Diagnosis and Medical Treatments

## 4.1 Visiting a Healthcare Professional

If you suspect you have gastritis or are experiencing symptoms of gastritis, it is essential to schedule a visit with a healthcare professional. A primary care physician or a gastroenterologist specializes in gastrointestinal disorders and can provide a comprehensive evaluation and diagnosis.

During your visit, the healthcare professional will review your medical history, including any symptoms you are experiencing, their duration, and any potential triggers or risk factors. They will also inquire about your diet, lifestyle habits, and any medications you are currently taking.

Be prepared to provide detailed information about your symptoms, including the location and severity of pain, any factors that worsen or alleviate the symptoms, and any associated symptoms like vomiting or changes in bowel habits. This information will help the healthcare professional make an accurate diagnosis and develop an appropriate treatment plan.

# 4.2 Diagnostic Tests for Gastritis

To confirm the diagnosis of gastritis and determine its underlying cause, the healthcare professional may recommend various diagnostic tests. These tests can help identify the presence of inflammation in the stomach lining and any contributing factors. Common diagnostic tests for gastritis include:

1.  Upper Endoscopy (Esophagogastroduodenoscopy or EGD): This procedure involves inserting a thin, flexible tube with a camera (endoscope) into the throat and down the esophagus to visualize the stomach and the first part of the small intestine. During the procedure, the healthcare professional can take biopsies (small tissue samples) of the

stomach lining to examine under a microscope for signs of inflammation, infection, or other abnormalities.

2.  Blood Tests: Blood tests can help identify markers of inflammation, such as elevated white blood cell counts or C-reactive protein levels. Blood tests may also be used to check for Helicobacter pylori infection or detect anemia, which may be associated with chronic gastritis.

3.  Stool Tests: Stool samples may be analyzed for the presence of Helicobacter pylori infection or to check for signs of blood loss in the digestive tract.

4.  Breath Test: A breath test can detect the presence of Helicobacter pylori by measuring the levels of

certain compounds in the breath after consuming a specific solution.

5. X-ray or CT Scan: These imaging studies may be used to identify structural abnormalities or complications associated with gastritis.

# 4.3 Conventional Medical Treatment Options

The treatment approach for gastritis will depend on its type (acute or chronic) and the underlying cause. Conventional medical treatment options for gastritis may include:

1. Acid-Suppressing Medications: Proton pump inhibitors (PPIs) or H2 receptor blockers are commonly prescribed to reduce

stomach acid production. These medications can provide relief from gastritis symptoms and promote healing of the stomach lining.

2.  Antibiotics: If Helicobacter pylori infection is detected, a combination of antibiotics is typically prescribed to eradicate the bacterium and reduce inflammation.

3.  Antacids: Over-the-counter antacids can provide temporary relief by neutralizing stomach acid and alleviating symptoms.

4.  Cytoprotective Agents: Medications that help protect the stomach lining, such as sucralfate, may be prescribed to promote healing.

5.  Lifestyle Modifications: The healthcare professional may recommend lifestyle changes, such as avoiding trigger foods, reducing alcohol and caffeine consumption, quitting smoking, and managing stress.

6.  Treatment for Underlying Conditions: If gastritis is caused by an underlying condition, such as autoimmune disorders or bile reflux, appropriate treatment for the underlying condition may be necessary.

It is essential to follow the healthcare professional's recommendations and complete the prescribed course of medications, even if symptoms improve. Additionally, lifestyle modifications, including dietary changes and stress management, can play a crucial role in supporting the healing process.

While conventional medical treatments can be effective in managing gastritis, it is essential to communicate openly with your healthcare professional about your symptoms and any concerns you may have. If you experience any adverse effects from medications or have questions about the treatment plan, do not hesitate to discuss them with your healthcare provider. In some cases, complementary therapies or alternative approaches may also be considered, but it is essential to consult with a healthcare professional before incorporating them into your treatment plan.

# CHAPTER 5

# Natural Approaches to Gastritis Healing

## 5.1 Lifestyle Changes for Gastritis Relief

Adopting certain lifestyle changes can significantly contribute to gastritis relief and support the healing process. Here are some lifestyle recommendations for managing gastritis:

1. Avoid Triggering Substances: Limit or avoid alcohol, caffeine, spicy foods, acidic foods, and carbonated beverages, as these can irritate the stomach lining and exacerbate gastritis symptoms.

2. Quit Smoking: Smoking can contribute to gastritis and delay healing. Quitting smoking can improve digestive health and reduce the risk of complications.

3. Eat Smaller and More Frequent Meals: Consuming smaller meals throughout the day rather than three large meals can help reduce the burden on the stomach and prevent excessive stomach acid production.

4. Maintain a Healthy Weight: Excess body weight can worsen gastritis symptoms. Aim to achieve and maintain a healthy weight through a balanced diet and regular exercise.

5. Practice Proper Posture: Avoid slouching or lying down immediately after eating. Maintain

good posture during and after meals to support proper digestion.

6. Avoid NSAIDs and Irritating Medications: If possible, avoid using nonsteroidal anti-inflammatory drugs (NSAIDs) or other medications that can irritate the stomach lining. Consult a healthcare professional for alternative pain relief options.

7. Get Adequate Sleep: Ensure you get enough restful sleep each night, as poor sleep can affect digestive health and exacerbate gastritis symptoms.

8. Stay Hydrated: Drink plenty of water throughout the day to maintain hydration and support digestive health.

## 5.2 Dietary Guidelines for Gastritis Healing

Adjusting your diet can play a vital role in healing gastritis and reducing symptoms. Here are some dietary guidelines for gastritis healing:

1. Consume a Gastritis-Friendly Diet: Choose foods that are gentle on the stomach, such as cooked vegetables, lean proteins (e.g., chicken, turkey, fish), whole grains, and low-fat dairy products.

2. Avoid Trigger Foods: Identify and avoid foods that trigger or worsen gastritis symptoms. Common triggers include spicy foods, acidic fruits, tomatoes, chocolate, coffee, and alcohol.

3. Incorporate Foods with Anti-Inflammatory Properties: Include

foods with anti-inflammatory properties in your diet, such as ginger, turmeric, garlic, and omega-3 fatty acids found in fatty fish like salmon.

4. Opt for Probiotics: Probiotics can support gut health and may help alleviate gastritis symptoms. Consider incorporating probiotic-rich foods like yogurt or fermented foods into your diet.

5. Chew Thoroughly: Chew your food thoroughly to aid digestion and reduce the workload on the stomach.

6. Avoid Overeating: Practice portion control to prevent overloading the stomach and minimize acid production.

7. Stay Hydrated: Drink water and herbal teas to stay hydrated and support digestion.

## 5.3 Herbal Remedies and Supplements

Certain herbal remedies and supplements may offer additional support for gastritis healing. However, it is essential to consult a healthcare professional before using any herbal remedies or supplements, especially if you are taking medications or have pre-existing health conditions. Some herbs and supplements that may be beneficial for gastritis include:

1. Aloe Vera: Aloe vera juice may help soothe the stomach lining and reduce inflammation.

2. Slippery Elm: Slippery elm can create a protective layer on the stomach lining and alleviate discomfort.

3. Chamomile: Chamomile tea is known for its calming and anti-inflammatory properties.

4. Licorice Root: Deglycyrrhizinated licorice (DGL) supplements may help protect the stomach lining and reduce inflammation.

5. Probiotics: Probiotic supplements can help restore a healthy balance of gut bacteria and promote digestive health.

Always follow the recommended dosage and guidelines provided by the supplement manufacturer or your healthcare professional.

# 5.4 Stress Management and Relaxation Techniques

Stress can exacerbate gastritis symptoms and delay healing. Implementing stress management and relaxation techniques can be beneficial. Consider the following approaches:

1.  Practice Mindfulness: Engage in mindfulness meditation or deep breathing exercises to reduce stress and promote relaxation.

2.  Yoga: Yoga combines physical postures, breathwork, and meditation, providing a holistic approach to stress reduction.

3.  Regular Exercise: Engaging in regular physical activity can help

reduce stress and support overall
well-being.

4. Get Enough Rest: Prioritize
   sufficient sleep and rest to allow
   the body to recover and heal.

5. Seek Emotional Support: Talk to
   friends, family, or a therapist about
   your concerns and emotions, as
   emotional support can help reduce
   stress.

6. Engage in Hobbies: Participate in
   activities you enjoy to distract
   from stress and promote
   relaxation.

By incorporating these natural
approaches into your lifestyle, you
can complement conventional medical
treatments and actively support the
healing of gastritis. Remember to
consult a healthcare professional
before making significant changes to

your diet, adding supplements, or starting a new exercise routine. They can provide personalized guidance based on your specific health needs and help you create a comprehensive approach to managing gastritis effectively.

# CHAPTER 6

# The Role of Nutrition in Gastritis Healing

## 6.1 Gastritis-Friendly Foods

Nutrition plays a vital role in gastritis healing, as certain foods can help soothe the stomach lining, reduce inflammation, and support the recovery process. Gastritis-friendly foods are typically easy on the stomach and less likely to trigger or worsen symptoms. Here are some examples of gastritis-friendly foods:

1. Cooked Vegetables: Steamed or boiled vegetables, such as carrots, zucchini, potatoes, and green beans, are easier to digest than raw vegetables.

2. Lean Proteins: Opt for lean proteins like skinless chicken, turkey, fish (e.g., salmon, cod), and tofu, as they are less likely to irritate the stomach.

3. Whole Grains: Choose whole grains like oats, rice, quinoa, and couscous, as they provide essential nutrients and fiber without putting excessive strain on the stomach.

4. Low-Fat Dairy: Consume low-fat dairy products, such as skim milk and low-fat yogurt, as they are less likely to trigger stomach discomfort.

5. Bananas: Bananas are gentle on the stomach and can provide essential nutrients and natural sugars.

6. Applesauce: Unsweetened applesauce is easy to digest and can be soothing for the stomach.

7. Oatmeal: Plain oatmeal is a good source of soluble fiber, which can be gentle on the digestive system.

8. Ginger: Ginger has natural anti-inflammatory properties and can be consumed as ginger tea or added to meals.

9. Herbal Teas: Chamomile, peppermint, and licorice root teas are known for their calming effects on the digestive system.

## 6.2 Foods to Avoid or Limit

Certain foods and beverages can exacerbate gastritis symptoms and delay healing. It is essential to avoid or limit these items to support gastritis recovery. Foods and beverages to avoid or limit include:

1. Spicy Foods: Avoid spicy dishes or ingredients like chili peppers and hot sauces, as they can irritate the stomach lining.

2. Acidic Foods: Citrus fruits (e.g., oranges, lemons, tomatoes) and acidic juices can worsen gastritis symptoms.

3. Coffee and Caffeinated Beverages: Coffee, tea, and caffeinated beverages can increase stomach

acid production and contribute to discomfort.

4. Alcohol: Alcohol can irritate the stomach lining and exacerbate gastritis symptoms. It is best to avoid alcohol during gastritis healing.

5. Carbonated Drinks: Carbonated beverages can lead to gas and bloating, which can be uncomfortable for those with gastritis.

6. Fatty and Fried Foods: High-fat and fried foods can slow down digestion and increase the risk of acid reflux.

7. Spicy Condiments: Spicy condiments like mustard, ketchup, and hot sauces should be used sparingly or avoided.

# 6.3 Meal Planning for Gastritis Relief

Meal planning is essential for managing gastritis and promoting healing. Here are some tips for planning meals that are gentle on the stomach:

1.  Eat Smaller, More Frequent Meals: Instead of large meals, aim for five to six smaller meals throughout the day to reduce the workload on the stomach.

2.  Chew Thoroughly: Take your time to chew food thoroughly to aid digestion and minimize stress on the stomach.

3.  Balance Macronutrients: Include a balance of carbohydrates, proteins,

and healthy fats in each meal to support overall nutrition.

4. Avoid Trigger Foods: Identify and avoid foods that trigger gastritis symptoms. Keep a food diary to track your reactions to different foods.

5. Incorporate Gastritis-Friendly Foods: Include cooked vegetables, lean proteins, whole grains, and gentle fruits in your meals.

6. Hydrate Wisely: Drink water and herbal teas between meals rather than with meals to prevent excessive stomach stretching.

7. Plan Snacks: Have gastritis-friendly snacks readily available, such as banana slices, plain crackers, or applesauce cups.

8. Avoid Late-Night Eating: Try to finish meals a few hours before bedtime to reduce the risk of acid reflux.

9. Plan Ahead: Prepare meals and snacks ahead of time to ensure you have gastritis-friendly options readily available.

10. Listen to Your Body: Pay attention to how your body responds to different foods and adjust your meal planning accordingly.

Individual tolerances to certain foods may vary, and what works for one person may not work for another. It is essential to work with a healthcare professional or a registered dietitian to create a personalized meal plan that meets your nutritional needs and supports gastritis healing effectively. A balanced and thoughtful approach to nutrition can play a significant role in managing gastritis and promoting digestive health.

# CHAPTER 7

# Home Remedies and Self-Care Practices

## 7.1 Soothing Teas and Drinks

Certain teas and drinks can provide soothing relief for gastritis symptoms and promote digestive health. Here are some soothing teas and drinks that may be beneficial:

1. Chamomile Tea: Chamomile has anti-inflammatory properties and

can help relax the digestive system. Sip on warm chamomile tea to soothe the stomach.

2. Ginger Tea: Ginger has natural anti-inflammatory effects and can help reduce nausea and stomach discomfort. Steep fresh ginger slices in hot water to make ginger tea.

3. Peppermint Tea: Peppermint can help ease indigestion and reduce bloating. Drink peppermint tea in moderation, as excessive consumption may worsen acid reflux in some individuals.

4. Licorice Root Tea: Licorice root tea may have a protective effect on the stomach lining and help reduce inflammation.

5. Warm Water with Honey: Sipping warm water with a teaspoon of

honey can provide gentle hydration and a soothing effect on the stomach.

6.  Aloe Vera Juice: Pure aloe vera juice can help soothe the stomach lining and reduce inflammation. Ensure it is free from additives or preservatives.

7.  Coconut Water: Coconut water is hydrating and may help replace electrolytes lost during vomiting or diarrhea.

Consume these beverages in moderation and listen to your body's response. While these teas and drinks can provide relief, excessive consumption may have adverse effects, especially if you have underlying health conditions.

## 7.2 Rest and Proper Sleep

Rest and sufficient sleep are crucial for the body's healing and recovery processes, including gastritis healing. Here are some tips for rest and proper sleep:

1. Prioritize Rest: Allow yourself adequate rest throughout the day, especially during periods of acute symptoms or flare-ups.

2. Create a Sleep-Friendly Environment: Make your sleeping environment conducive to rest by keeping the room cool, dark, and quiet. Invest in a comfortable mattress and pillows.

3. Establish a Sleep Routine: Try to go to bed and wake up at the

same time each day to regulate
your body's sleep-wake cycle.

4. Limit Screen Time Before Bed:
   Avoid screens (e.g., phones,
   computers, TVs) at least an
   hour before bedtime, as the
   blue light can disrupt sleep.

5. Practice Relaxation
   Techniques: Engage in
   relaxation practices like deep
   breathing, meditation, or gentle
   stretching before bedtime to
   calm the mind and body.

6. Limit Stimulants: Avoid
   consuming caffeine or other
   stimulants close to bedtime, as
   they can interfere with sleep.

7. Limit Late-Night Eating: Finish
   your meals a few hours before
   bedtime to reduce the risk of

acid reflux and improve sleep quality.

Proper rest and sleep not only aid in gastritis healing but also contribute to overall well-being. When experiencing gastritis symptoms, listen to your body and allow yourself the necessary rest for optimal recovery.

While these home remedies and self-care practices can provide relief and support healing, it's important to remember that they should not replace professional medical advice or treatment. If you have severe or persistent symptoms, consult a healthcare professional for proper evaluation and management. They can offer personalized recommendations and ensure you receive the most appropriate care for your specific condition.

# CHAPTER 8

# Understanding the Gut-Brain Connection

## 8.1 The Gut-Brain Axis

The gut-brain axis is a bidirectional communication network between the gastrointestinal system (the gut) and the brain. This complex system involves a constant exchange of signals and information between the two, influencing various physiological and psychological processes. The gut and the brain are connected through the nervous system, hormonal pathways, and immune system. The gut is often referred to as the "second brain" due to the extensive network of neurons in the gut, known as the enteric nervous system.

The gut-brain axis plays a crucial role in various aspects of human health, including digestion, mood regulation, immune function, and even cognitive processes. For example:

1.  Digestion and Appetite Regulation: The brain sends signals to the gut, affecting digestion, nutrient absorption, and appetite. Additionally, the gut communicates with the brain to signal feelings of hunger or satiety.

2. Emotional Regulation: The gut produces neurotransmitters such as serotonin, often referred to as the "happy hormone." Serotonin plays a significant role in regulating mood, emotions, and overall well-being.

3. Stress Response: The gut-brain axis is intimately involved in the body's stress response. Stress can affect gut function and vice versa, leading to gastrointestinal issues.

4. Immune Function: The gut houses a significant portion of the body's immune cells and plays a crucial role in immune system regulation. Communication between the gut and the brain influences immune responses to infections and inflammation.

## 8.2 Mindful Eating for Gastritis Healing

Mindful eating is a practice that encourages awareness and presence while consuming food. It involves paying attention to the sensory experiences of eating, such as taste, texture, and aroma, as well as tuning into hunger and fullness cues. Mindful eating can be beneficial for individuals with gastritis as it can help manage symptoms and promote healing. Here are some tips for mindful eating:

1. Eat Without Distractions: Avoid eating while watching TV, using electronic devices, or engaging in other distracting activities. Focus solely on your meal.

2. Chew Slowly: Take your time to chew food thoroughly before

swallowing. Chewing well aids digestion and can reduce strain on the stomach.

3. Pay Attention to Hunger and Fullness: Tune in to your body's hunger and fullness cues. Eat when you're hungry and stop when you feel satisfied.

4. Savor the Flavors: Appreciate the taste and flavors of your food. Mindfully experience each bite.

5. Be Present: Bring your attention to the present moment during meals. Avoid rushing or multitasking while eating.

6. Listen to Your Body: Be attentive to how different foods make you feel. Notice if certain foods trigger or alleviate gastritis symptoms.

Practicing mindful eating can help improve digestion and reduce the likelihood of overeating, which can be beneficial for individuals with gastritis.

# CHAPTER 9

# Gastritis and Stress Management

## 9.1 How Stress Impacts Gastritis

Stress can have a significant impact on gastritis and digestive health. When you experience stress, the body enters a "fight or flight" response, triggering the release of stress hormones like cortisol and adrenaline.

This physiological response can affect various aspects of digestion:

1. Increased Stomach Acid: Stress can stimulate the production of stomach acid, which can irritate the stomach lining and worsen gastritis symptoms.

2. Reduced Blood Flow to the Gut: During periods of stress, blood flow is redirected away from the digestive system to support other functions, potentially leading to digestive issues.

3. Altered Gut Motility: Stress can affect gut motility, leading to symptoms like bloating, gas, and changes in bowel movements.

4. Impact on Gut Microbiota: Stress may influence the composition of the gut microbiota, which can affect gut health and inflammation.

## 9.2 Stress-Relief Techniques

Managing stress is essential for individuals with gastritis to support healing and prevent symptom exacerbation. Here are some stress-relief techniques that may be beneficial:

1. Meditation: Regular meditation practices, such as mindfulness meditation or guided imagery, can help calm the mind and reduce stress.

2. Deep Breathing Exercises: Deep breathing techniques can activate the body's relaxation response and promote a sense of calm.

3. Yoga: Yoga combines physical postures, breathwork, and

meditation, providing a holistic
approach to stress reduction.

4. Exercise: Regular physical
   activity, such as walking, jogging,
   or swimming, can help reduce
   stress and promote overall well-
   being.

5. Journaling: Keeping a journal to
   express emotions, thoughts, and
   concerns can be a helpful way to
   process stress.

6. Social Support: Connect with
   friends, family, or support groups
   to share experiences and receive
   emotional support.

7. Time Management: Organize tasks
   and prioritize responsibilities to
   reduce feelings of overwhelm and
   stress.

8. Mindfulness Practices: Engage in activities that promote mindfulness, such as spending time in nature, listening to music, or practicing a creative hobby.

9. Seek Professional Help: If stress becomes overwhelming or difficult to manage on your own, consider speaking with a mental health professional or counselor.

By incorporating stress-relief techniques into daily life, individuals with gastritis can positively influence the gut-brain axis and promote overall digestive health. Reducing stress can complement medical treatments and support the body's natural healing processes for gastritis.

# CHAPTER 10

# Incorporating Exercise into Your Healing Journey

# 10.1 Exercise and Gastritis Relief

Incorporating regular exercise into your healing journey can be beneficial for managing gastritis and promoting overall well-being. While intense or high-impact exercises may not be suitable during acute gastritis flare-ups, moderate and low-impact physical activities can offer numerous benefits:

1. Stress Reduction: Exercise can help reduce stress levels, which is particularly important as stress can exacerbate gastritis symptoms.

2. Improved Digestion: Regular physical activity can support healthy digestion and bowel movements.

3. Weight Management: Maintaining a healthy weight can help reduce pressure on the stomach and lower the risk of acid reflux.

4. Enhanced Blood Circulation: Exercise improves blood flow, which can support the healing of inflamed tissues in the stomach lining.

5. Mood Enhancement: Engaging in physical activity can trigger the release of endorphins, promoting a positive mood and overall sense of well-being.

6. Immune System Support: Regular exercise can boost the immune system, aiding in the body's ability to fight infections, including those related to gastritis.

## 10.2 Choosing the Right Physical Activities

When selecting physical activities during your healing journey, it's essential to consider your current health status and the severity of your gastritis symptoms. Here are some guidelines for choosing the right exercises:

1. Low-Impact Activities: Opt for low-impact exercises to minimize strain on the stomach and joints. Walking, swimming, cycling, and gentle yoga are excellent options.

2. Listen to Your Body: Pay attention to how your body responds to different exercises. If an activity causes discomfort or worsens symptoms, consider choosing a gentler option.

3. Avoid Strenuous Workouts During Flare-Ups: During acute gastritis flare-ups, it's best to avoid intense or high-impact workouts. Focus on rest and gentle movements until symptoms subside.

4. Gradual Progression: If you are new to exercise or have been inactive for a while, start with gentle activities and gradually increase intensity and duration as your body adapts.

5. Warm-Up and Cool Down: Always warm up before exercising to prepare your body for physical activity, and cool down afterward to ease your body back to a resting state.

6. Hydration: Stay well-hydrated before, during, and after exercise,

as proper hydration supports digestion and overall health.

7. Consult Your Healthcare Professional: Before starting a new exercise routine, especially if you have underlying health conditions or concerns, consult your healthcare professional to ensure it is safe and suitable for you.

Everyone's tolerance for exercise is different, so it's essential to find activities that work best for you and your healing journey. Consistency is key, but be gentle with yourself and allow your body time to recover and heal. If you experience any adverse reactions or symptoms during or after exercising, consult your healthcare professional for guidance.

# CHAPTER 11

# Maintaining Gastritis Healing Long-Term

## 11.1 Preventive Measures

Maintaining gastritis healing long-term involves adopting preventive measures to minimize the risk of gastritis recurrence and promote overall digestive health. By incorporating these practices into your daily life, you can support the healing process and reduce the likelihood of gastritis flare-ups:

1. Follow a Gastritis-Friendly Diet: Continue to eat a balanced diet that is gentle on the stomach, incorporating cooked vegetables, lean proteins, whole grains, and low-fat dairy products. Avoid trigger foods that may exacerbate gastritis symptoms.

2. Stay Hydrated: Drink plenty of water and herbal teas to maintain

hydration and support healthy digestion.

3. Avoid Excessive Alcohol and Caffeine: Limit or avoid alcohol and caffeinated beverages, as they can irritate the stomach lining and contribute to gastritis.

4. Quit Smoking: If you smoke, consider quitting to support gastric healing and overall well-being.

5. Manage Stress: Practice stress-relief techniques, such as meditation, deep breathing, yoga, or engaging in hobbies, to minimize stress levels.

6. Exercise Regularly: Incorporate regular physical activity into your routine, choosing low-impact exercises that suit your health status.

7. Practice Mindful Eating: Continue to eat mindfully, paying attention to hunger and fullness cues and savoring the flavors of your food.

8. Limit NSAIDs and Irritating Medications: Avoid using nonsteroidal anti-inflammatory drugs (NSAIDs) or other medications that can irritate the stomach lining unless prescribed by your healthcare professional.

9. Maintain a Healthy Weight: Aim to achieve and maintain a healthy weight through a balanced diet and regular exercise.

10. Get Adequate Sleep: Prioritize sufficient restful sleep to support healing and overall well-being.

11. Follow Medical Recommendations: Continue to follow your healthcare

professional's recommendations regarding medication, treatment, and follow-up visits.

12. Monitor Your Symptoms: Be aware of any changes or new symptoms and promptly consult your healthcare professional if you experience recurrent or worsening gastritis symptoms.

13. Manage Underlying Health Conditions: If you have underlying health conditions that contribute to gastritis, work with your healthcare professional to manage and treat these conditions effectively.

14. Avoid Overeating and Late-Night Eating: Practice portion control and avoid eating late at night to reduce the risk of acid reflux and digestive discomfort.

15. Regular Check-Ups: Schedule regular check-ups with your healthcare professional to monitor your gastritis healing progress and overall digestive health.

Individual responses to preventive measures may vary, and it's essential to listen to your body and adapt your lifestyle as needed. By incorporating these preventive measures into your daily routine, you can support long-term gastritis healing and enjoy improved digestive health and well-being. If you have any concerns or questions, always consult your healthcare professional for personalized guidance and advice.

# 11.2 Monitoring Your Gastritis Progress

Monitoring your gastritis progress is essential to assess the effectiveness of your healing journey and make any necessary adjustments to your treatment and lifestyle. Here are some tips on how to monitor your gastritis progress:

1. Keep a Symptom Diary: Maintain a daily or weekly journal to track your gastritis symptoms, including the type and severity of pain, frequency of flare-ups, and any triggers you notice. This can help you identify patterns and potential triggers for your symptoms.

2. Record Dietary Intake: Note your daily food intake in your symptom diary. Keep track of any specific foods that seem to worsen or

improve your symptoms. This can help you identify foods that may be contributing to gastritis and make informed dietary choices.

3. Assess Stress Levels: Monitor your stress levels regularly. Stress can impact gastritis symptoms, so keeping track of stress triggers and how you respond to stress-reduction techniques can be valuable.

4. Track Medication and Treatment: If you are on medication or following a specific treatment plan, keep a record of your medication schedule and any changes in treatment. Note how you respond to medications and any side effects you experience.

5. Observe Sleep Quality: Pay attention to the quality and

duration of your sleep. Poor sleep can exacerbate gastritis symptoms, so aim to improve your sleep habits if necessary.

6. Check for Recurring Symptoms: Watch out for recurring symptoms or new symptoms that may indicate a flare-up or complications. If you notice any concerning changes, consult your healthcare professional.

7. Schedule Follow-Up Visits: Regularly schedule follow-up visits with your healthcare professional to discuss your progress, review your symptom diary, and make any necessary adjustments to your treatment plan.

8. Evaluate Lifestyle Changes: Assess how well you have been implementing lifestyle changes,

such as dietary modifications, exercise, stress reduction, and mindful eating. Identify areas for improvement and make gradual adjustments to your habits.

9.  Seek Support: If you have any concerns or questions, don't hesitate to reach out to your healthcare professional for guidance and support. They can offer personalized advice based on your specific condition and progress.

10. Celebrate Achievements: Recognize and celebrate the positive changes you've made on your healing journey. Acknowledge the progress you've made in managing gastritis and continue to stay motivated to maintain a healthy lifestyle.

By actively monitoring your gastritis progress, you can identify what works best for you and make informed decisions about your health and well-being. Remember that healing takes time, and it's essential to be patient and persistent in your efforts. With consistent monitoring and support from your healthcare professional, you can optimize your gastritis healing and maintain a healthier lifestyle in the long term.

# CHAPTER 12

# Signs of Improvement

Knowing when to reevaluate your gastritis healing progress is crucial to ensure you are on the right track and to make any necessary adjustments to your treatment plan. Here are some signs of improvement that may indicate it's time for a reevaluation:

1.  Decreased Frequency and Severity of Symptoms: If you notice a reduction in the frequency and severity of gastritis symptoms, such as abdominal pain, bloating, nausea, or indigestion, it could be a sign of improvement.

2. Better Tolerance of Trigger Foods: If you find that you can tolerate certain foods that previously triggered gastritis symptoms, it may indicate an improvement in the health of your stomach lining.

3. Improved Quality of Life: Feeling more comfortable and experiencing an overall improvement in your quality of life, including better sleep, improved mood, and increased energy levels, can be positive indicators.

4. Successful Tapering of Medications: If you have been on medications for gastritis, successfully tapering off or reducing the dosage under the guidance of your healthcare

professional may suggest healing progress.

5. Regularity in Digestive Patterns: If you notice more regular bowel movements and improved digestion, it can be a sign of better gastrointestinal health.

6. Reduced Reliance on Acid-Suppressing Medications: If you were previously dependent on acid-suppressing medications for symptom relief and find that you need them less frequently, it could be a positive sign.

7. Ability to Resume Regular Activities: If you can resume regular activities, including exercise and social engagements, without

significant gastritis-related limitations, it may indicate progress.

It's essential to maintain open communication with your healthcare professional throughout your healing journey. They can provide guidance, assess your progress, and make any necessary adjustments to your treatment plan based on your individual needs and responses. Regular follow-up visits and proactive discussions can help optimize your gastritis healing and overall digestive health.